ADVENTUROUS

POEMS THAT WILL BOOST YOUR SELF-ESTEEM

UDO EBULU

DEDICATION

I dedicate this book to my younger cousin, Olaedo Igbo. Your ambition, optimism, and beautiful soul inspires me to continue to be ambitious and optimistic.

TABLE OF CONTENTS

INTRODUCTION

"Aye! She's in my psychology class. She is *sexy*." That's what I said to myself when I noticed her on campus. I remember it like it was yesterday. It was my first semester freshman year of college. I walked to my 9:00 am psychology class to wait in the classroom 30 minutes early. What a nerd right? That's when I saw her. The sight of her beauty stopped me in my tracks. A part of me said to myself, "This is your chance, go talk to her." Another part of me said, "I'm scared, she might reject me." I noticed that she saw me too, so I had to decide quickly. I said to myself, "You can do this Udoka, c'mon." So I continued to make my move, faster than usual. My heart was racing, I was scared. But I kept saying to myself, "You can do this Udoka." I was thinking of a pick-up line. Something like, "Aye girl, are you from Tennessee? Because you're the only ten I see."

The moment arrived. As soon as I got close, I said to her in a quiet voice, "Hey how you doing?" as I walked right past her. I glanced into her eyes. She waved and softly replied, "Hi." Unfortunately, my low self-esteem got the best of that moment.

How we value ourselves strongly influence our health, motivation, relationships, and overall quality of life. Having low self-esteem can lead to mental health issues, inability to pursue goals, and unhealthy relationships. Low self-esteem may manifest in a variety of ways, often beginning in childhood. This is either from experiences of fear, being bullied, or worries of insecurities.

Having high self-esteem can lead to good health, healthy relationships, and self-fulfillment. To have high self-esteem means knowing who you are, expressing yourself freely, and having confidence in your abilities.

I had such low self-esteem as a teenager that I became reserved.

So reserved, that days after my 18th birthday, I looked over my life and was highly disappointed in myself. As a result, I used the beginning of my adulthood as an opportunity to restart my life, improve my self-esteem, and be more, *Adventurous.*

There have been times when I've tried and failed. But through those failures I learned what I did wrong. Then I tried again until I succeeded. Since then, I've become a risk-taker. I am now more successful, and I will continue to succeed in life. I refuse to be that shy, conservative teenager ever again. I'd rather try and fail than not try at all.

I've written several self-esteem-boosting poems about the concept of fear, being yourself, and focusing on the positives in life. I compiled that and more in the pages of this book. If poetry interests you and you want to improve your self-esteem, this book is for you.

Now that we have gotten the introduction out of the way, let's get into the first chapter, Empowerment.

Chapter 1: Empowerment

The process of growing stronger and more confident while taking control of one's life.

Talking to Myself

"If you know better, do better," is what I say to myself.
Why do anything that's not good for my health?
A career with passion, why choose anything else?
I ought to be patient and work for long-term wealth.
"Patience is a virtue," is what I try to remember,
any and every year, January to December.
The best things happen to those who wait.
Don't settle for good, strive to be great.
"Greatness is within you," I say to my reflection.
Focus on you, pay yourself attention.
Understand that you are not above correction,
and aim for the stars, the bullseye, perfection.

Check This Out

If I say I'll do something, best believe I'll do it.
Once I set it in my mind, there isn't anything to it.
I go over it thoroughly, then I make the decision.
Most people have eyes, but few people have vision.
I'm not scared to fail and I'm not scared to fall,
because before I could walk, I first had to crawl.
I hate it when I lose, but I never ever stop trying,
because in those losses I learn, then I start frying.
When I set my mind to something, I'll always do my best,
in all that I can control, and let God handle the rest.

Earn It

God helps those that help themselves.
Gilt-edged knowledge, found in bookshelves.
Having time does not mean to procrastinate.
Stall long enough and it will be too late.
Less is more, call it reverse-abundance.
Walk and talk out of an adverse circumstance.
Greatness is synonymous with responsibility.
It's up to you to make your dream a reality.

Chapter 2: Encouragement

The act of giving support, hope, or confidence
to another person.

The Journey

The best things in life do not come easy.
If this is fiction, life would be breezy.
This is not to say, it's not worth fighting for.
You have accomplished a lot, yet still so many more,
goals to set, and goals to obtain,
trying to achieve them without going insane.
When things go wrong, don't go with them.
Dig deep inside for that hidden gem,
that's within your heart and within your soul,
amid all the darkness, a sudden glow,
at the end of the tunnel, can you see the light?
Letting you know, it will be alright.

Passion & Desire

An electric vibe, a burning sensation.
All through the year, not just an occasion.
Outside I'm cool, inside I'm warm.
Out of touch most times, little time for the norm.
Brings me joy, gives me purpose.
Boosts my confidence, especially when nervous.
All about that action, I play with fire.
It's because of my passion, and my desire.

Do Yourself a Favor

Be you, no one else will do it better.
Be bold, write yourself a love letter.
Worry less about fitting in, feel free to stand out.
Chasing your dreams is cooler than chasing clout.
The road to happiness starts from within.
It's about finding comfort in your own skin.
He say, she say, who cares what they say.
The key say is your say. Live your life, your way.

Chapter 3: Enlightenment

The state of having great knowledge or understanding about a subject or situation.

Fear

A troubling feeling triggered by a perceived danger,
in the form of uncertainty or a complete stranger.
Physical, mental, and emotional distress,
all the makings of an enemy of progress.
Real or imagined this feeling should not,
stop you from wanting to earn the top spot,
of your dreams, and goals, and heart's desire.
Rather provide you clarity, and fuel your fire.

Truth Is

Truth is, truth hurts, that's the truth.
Not all truth is bad, I'll provide proof.
People won't tell you there's something in your tooth,
smiling and what not, before you enter the booth.
In the photo, contrary to what you've heard,
there's not just a dental flaw, and no one said a word.
If one person, just one person spoke on the fact,
would you have been receptive or take it as an attack?
Truth is, truth hurts, that's the truth.
Not all truth is bad, don't be aloof.

Bullies

Let me tell you,
I crush bullies,
I crush them good.
Chew them up,
spit them out,
I wish a bully would.
They pick on those that they believe to be small,
to compensate deep down for being two feet tall.
They'll do anything to make them feel superior,
and hide the traits that make them feel inferior.
Bullies bully because they are dense, immature,
mentally ill, traumatized, miserable, insecure.
In a school, in the home, the workplace, or online,
what goes around comes around, all in due time.

Chapter 4: Enjoyment

A state or process of finding pleasure in something.

I Am An Artist

I am an artist, I live through my art.
All different kinds come from my heart.
I love to create, I love how it feels.
I can't really explain, it's just so surreal.
Every day I tap out of reality,
and into a world of originality.
I've been told that I'm crazy, I understand why.
People don't understand me, they don't even try.
Art is my life, I need to be crazy,
because if I'm not, then I would be lazy.
It's the gift I was given, art is my passion.
It brings me joy, and satisfaction.

The Elephant in Me

Just like an elephant, my extraordinary memory,
is one of the many traits of the elephant in me.
Their resiliency is a sign of their extraordinary strength.
Their loyalty to loved ones goes to an extreme length.
Compassionately fierce, they will do anything to protect,
their family from harm their intuition can detect.
Optimism is probably their most endearing quality.
They symbolize good news, good vibes, and prosperity.

The Good in My Life

With all the bad in my life that makes me sore,
there is also good to be grateful for.
Like the parents that God has given to me,
and the siblings, so grateful he gave me three.
To the people that show me unconditional support,
my appreciation goes beyond the verbal sort.
Thankful for my talents, skills, and abilities,
my cup overflows with glorious possibilities.
For the experiences that formulate my attitude,
the good and the bad, I have nothing but gratitude.

Chapter 5: Bonus

God Willing

I will make life easier for those around me.
That is, my friends and family.
A difference that will create more unity.

I will explore the world beyond the present me,
to see all that I'm allowed to see.
Understand what others wish that their life could be.

I will outduel those plotting against me,
be it a supposed ally or a blatant enemy.
Only God and me will rule my destiny.

My Personal Prayer

Lord, I'm a perfectionist, human beings are not perfect.
My standards are high, greatness is what I expect.
I pray that when I make mistakes in the future,
they'll be new and honest, to learn from, like a tutor.

Aww Mmu

A student of life, a king at heart.
Modest and kind, top of the chart.
More than capable of leading a nation.
Able to adapt to any situation.
Highly dedicated to accomplishing a goal.
Rich in the mind, body, and soul.
Magnificent style, magnificent flow.
Star of the sky, star of the show.
I am the one with the eccentric point of view.
I am Udo Ebulu. That's right, Aww Mmu!

EPILOGUE

"What is wrong with me?" That's what I asked myself as soon as I was out of her sight. "You promised to not be shy and conservative ever again. You are Udoka! Turn around and go talk to her NOW!" Thanks to my self-motivation, I courageously turned around. I had no idea what I was going to say. I just knew that I had to, and was *going* to say something.

I walked over to her and gently asked, "Hey, we have psychology class together right?" She answered, "Yes, we do." Then I asked, "Were you able to finish the homework assignment?" She replied, "No, I missed class. What did we have to do?" I sat beside her and explained the assignment.

I told her my name when she asked, she did the same when I asked for hers. She was so enthusiastic while talking to me, it felt like she wanted me to come talk to her. I'm glad that I did. We walked together to our class, sat beside each other, and the rest, is history.

The sense of value that we have for ourselves play a vital role in our health, motivation, relationships, and lives in general. Low self-esteem creates mental health problems, obstacles in achieving goals, and toxicity in relationships. Having high self-esteem is being comfortable in your own skin, speaking willingly, and believing in yourself.

It is important to find a healthy balance of self-esteem. Self-esteem that is too high may give a sense of entitlement. This can be detrimental to personal growth. Some indications of healthy self-esteem are confidence (not cockiness), respect for yourself and to others, and acceptance of your strengths and weaknesses.

I hope that you enjoyed reading this book and learned valuable lessons from it. I hope that this book helps boost your self-esteem and make you more, *Adventurous!*

ACKNOWLEDGMENTS

To the man upstairs, heavenly father, king of kings, lord of lords, alpha and omega, almighty God! Thank you! It is because of you and your blessings that this book came to life.

I would also like to thank my awesome editor and consultant, T. Marie Bell, best-selling author of "I Heard God's Voice." Your professional advice and guidance towards this book cannot be overstated.

My wonderful mother, Clara Igbo. I love your fun spirit, strong work-ethic, encouragement, love and support, all of it! You're the best, thank you mommy!

My precious sister, Ujunwa "Asanwa" Ebulu. Thank you for your generosity, and for being there for me whenever I get myself into trouble.

My Irish twin brother, Ifeanyi "Chuku100" Ebulu. Thank you for your shout-outs, and challenging me to become a better version of myself.

My oil slick brother, Obinna "Oil Slick" Ebulu. Thank you for your understanding, and helping me to remain optimistic with your enthusiasm.

Thank you Chena Johnson, for believing in me and inspiring me to write this book in the first place. You are wonderful!

My guy Chukwuemeka "Chuck" Nwapora, author of "From the Hood to Hollywood". Thank you also for believing in me. Your selfless efforts towards this book are invaluable. You're a boss for real!

Scribe Media, you had the answers to all of my questions for my book and more. Thank you for all of your phenomenal advice!

My supporters, oh my goodness! My heart aches for this part because I don't want to leave anyone out. I am speaking to you from the bottom of my heart. Thank you so much for your genuine love. Thank you for all of the support shown. From your kind words, to kind gestures, I am forever grateful!

ABOUT THE AUTHOR

Udo Ebulu took a leap of faith and relocated from Prince George's County, Maryland to Atlanta, Georgia in 2020. On a wing and prayer, without employment or a support system in place, Udo moved cross country to take his film career to the next level.

Currently, Udo resides in Atlanta, Georgia where he recently produced a crime, drama, mystery film titled, *"It Wasn't Me"*. He also modeled in fashion runway shows presented by Streetwear Fashion Week.

Thank you for supporting Mr. Ebulu's book *"Adventurous"*! He greatly appreciates it!

You may contact him at:
udoebulu@peaceisbetterentertainment.com

www.ingramcontent.com/pod-product-compliance
Lightning Source LLC
LaVergne TN
LVHW041239080426
835508LV00011B/1279